The Yin and Yang
of
Aging

The Yin and Yang
of
Aging

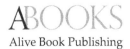

Ted Fuller

Cartoons by Barry Hunau

ABOOKS
Alive Book Publishing

Additional copies may be ordered from the publisher for educational,
business, promotional or premium use.
For information, contact ALIVE Book Publishing at:
alivebookpublishing.com, or call (925) 837-7303.

Book Design by Alex Johnson

ISBN 13
978-1-63132-034-7

ISBN 10
1-63132-034-3

Library of Congress Control Number: 2016943688
Library of Congress Cataloging-in-Publication Data is available upon request.

First Edition

Published in the United States of America by ALIVE Book Publishing
and ALIVE Publishing Group, imprints of Advanced Publishing LLC
3200 A Danville Blvd., Suite 204, Alamo, California 94507
alivebookpublishing.com

PRINTED IN THE UNITED STATES OF AMERICA

10 9 8 7 6 5 4 3 2 1

Acknowledgments

Many of these segments first appeared in *Senior Solutions*, a newsletter published by the Diablo Valley Foundation for the Aging in Walnut Creek, California, and are reprinted here with its permission.

Barry Hunau practiced dentistry for thirty-eight years, then started a second career as an editorial cartoonist. His cartoons have appeared in newspapers here and abroad. He illustrated two books and has created numerous posters for local theatrical productions. When time permits, he acts in some of them.

Table of Contents

Foreword

Tips on aging are scattered all over the Internet, the library, television, newspapers, and magazines. This book includes some of the key elements in concise form enhanced by the humorous cartoons of Barry Hunau and jokes or sayings that shine a different shade of light on things.

And, why, you may ask, the "yin and yang"?

According to a Chinese theory, yin is the passive, negative force, and yang the active, positive force. According to this theory, wise people will detect these forces in the seasons, in their food, and so on, and regulate their lives accordingly.

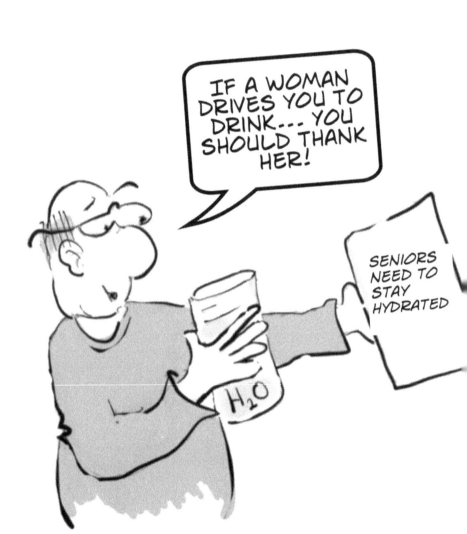

A habit worth having

W.C. Fields once remarked, "I never drink water-that's the stuff that rusts pipes." He also said that the reason he didn't drink it was it might become habit forming. The comedian got lots of laughs with thoughts like these, but, when it comes to water, he was, pardon the expression, all wet.

Folks who are aging should especially disregard Mr. Fields, according to Dr. Deepak Chopra. "Not drinking enough water every day is one of the commonest conditions in old age, and, although it has received almost no publicity, chronic dehydration is a major cause of preventable aging," he says. In *Ageless Body, Timeless Mind,* he notes, "Some authorities go so far as to count dehydration among the leading causes of death in old age."

Without enough water, difficulties such as kidney failure, heart problems, dizziness, lethargy, and senile dementia can occur. It can lead to a vicious circle. A person becomes forgetful about drinking water, then has difficulty seeing the problem. Often he or she becomes depressed.

Some depressed seniors turn to alcohol. If they're also taking drugs, the problems multiply. Other older people may withdraw, become isolated.

As for W.C. Fields, he played a distrustful, hard-drinking egotist with great contempt for children and dogs. He started as a juggler in vaudeville, incorporated comedy in his act, and starred in the Ziegfeld Follies. Among his observations:

I never drink water because of the disgusting things that fish do in it.

Anyone who hates children and animals can't be all bad.

On days you feel flat

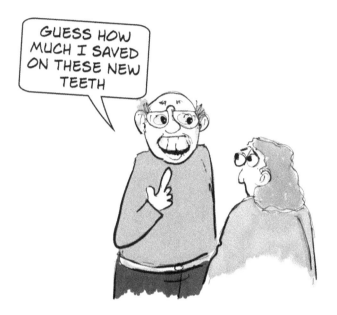

In *The Joys of Aging & How to Avoid Them,* Phyllis Diller wonders, "If I found the Fountain of Youth [and] just went in up to my toes, would I end up with young feet?"

Changes that come with age aren't a laughing matter for some folks. The loss of loved ones, physical challenges, or loneliness may cause emotional stress.

"The diagnosis of depression in older adults is often missed," says Moira Fordyce, M.D. "The person may deny sadness, and the health practitioner might not think to elicit more information from the sufferer, or his or her partner, about such important symptoms as loss of interest in previously enjoyed pastimes."

"The death of a loved one may cause grieving and sadness, which are normal reactions," says Dr. Fordyce, a Stanford University School of Medicine professor. "Most people, in due course, are able to get on with their lives." For some, however, the grieving tips over into depression.

Factors such as medications also may affect mood and memory. The use of alcohol and other substances also must be considered, she says. People with depression can be helped, but it takes accurate diagnoses and prompt treatment.

On a visit to her psychiatrist, Phyllis Diller promptly unloaded her troubles. Finally he said, "You're crazy."

"I'd like another opinion," she said.

"Okay," he said, "you're also ugly."

It's time to begin

Motivational speaker Marsha Doble admits, "I have to exercise early in the morning, before my brain figures out what the hell I'm doing." Anthropologists explain one reason some of us resist exercise. It's called "The Principles of Least Effort." They define it thus: "Any creature, when having a task to perform, will select the way of performing the task that requires the least effort."

In his book, *Living Longer for Dummies*, Dr. Walter Bortz notes that we're exploiting that principle to a high degree. "Look at the golf cart, electric carving knife, and electric toothbrush. At this rate, our poor muscles will have nothing left to do."

He emphasizes that "Exercise for the young is an option, but exercise for the old is a must."

The elderly must build and maintain their health reserves, and the key to achieving them is exercise. "People don't stop moving when they get old," he says. "People get old when they stop moving."

He serves as an excellent example of the plus side of exercise. Devastated in 1973 by the death of his father, who also was a doctor, he floundered and became depressed. "Then I started to run in a desperate effort to escape my grief. It worked." Dr. Bortz has run a marathon every year since, and added weight lifting and stretching to his routine in 1998.

"If we opt for sloth, we run increased risks of cardiovascular vulnerability, musculoskelatal fragility, immunologic susceptibility, obesity, depression, and premature aging," he says. "A fit person of 70 corresponds biologically to an unfit person of 40."

He likes to quote jazz pianist Eubie Blake, who said, "I'd have taken better care of myself if I had known I would live this long." Then the doctor adds for those of us who have skipped exercise for several decades, "Starting late is better than never starting at all."

In the book she co-authored with her sister Bessie, Sadie Delany said, "You've got to exercise, not just for your heart and lungs, but to keep from stiffening up. It keeps you limber, and that's important when you get older." She expressed her views in *The Delany Sisters' Book of Everyday Wisdom*. It came out when they were 105 and 103 years old, respectively. "We started doing yoga about forty years ago," Sadie said. "When we were younger and lived in New York City, we'd walk for miles because we couldn't afford to take the trolley. That was mighty good exercise!"

She died at the age of 109 in 1999, four years after Bessie died at 104.

Opportunities Missed

There was a very cautious man
Who never laughed or played.
He never risked, he never tried,
He never sang or prayed.
And when he one day passed away
His insurance was denied,
For since he never really lived
They claimed he never died.

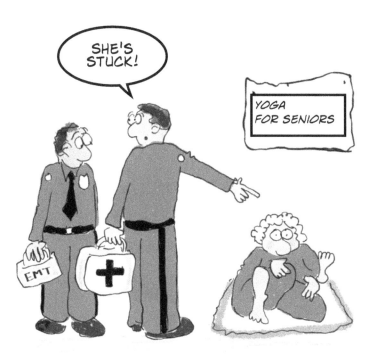

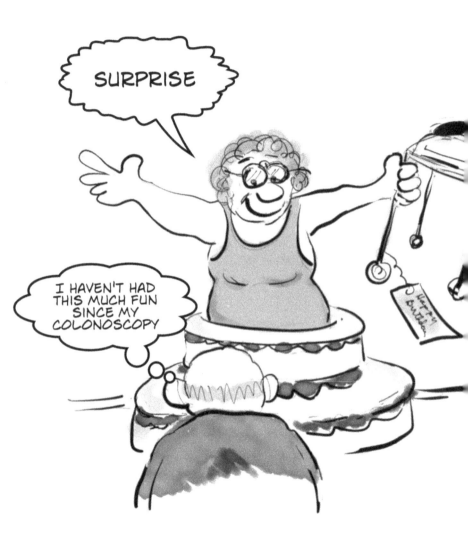

An example of bravery

An ailing friend once wrote Mark Twain, "Could there be anything worse than having a toothache and an earache at the same time?"

He wrote back: "Rheumatism and St. Vitus' dance."

Agencies that assist older adults find that their clients often experience double whammies comparable to Mark Twain's rejoinder. The eighty-seven-year-old woman, who no longer can drive, discovers that the nephew who drives her places also is siphoning money from her checking account. Another example: a recently retired man with diabetes fractures a hip after falling.

It takes bravery along with help from concerned outsiders to cope with such disasters. Clara Barton, founder of the American Red Cross at the age of sixty, provides an example of tenacity, help, and courage. Once described as "timid as a mouse, but brave as a lion," she continued to fulfill her destiny as the years rolled by.

In her earlier years, she became a teacher when mostly men were chosen in that field. After the Civil War began, she risked her life to take supplies and provide help to men in the field. With the Red Cross, Barton journeyed wherever turmoil led to harm and danger. She and her associates provided relief following fires, earthquakes, floods, and conflicts. During the Spanish-American war in 1898, she served in Cuba after she'd turned seventy-seven.

Barton resigned as Red Cross president and founded the National First Aid Association and served as its president for five years. During her lifetime she helped bring about positive changes in education, prison reform, the women's suffragette movement, and civil rights. She died in 1912 at the age of ninety-one.

On one occasion, an associate asked Barton about an insult that occurred years earlier. She maintained that it hadn't happened.

"Don't you remember it?"

"No," she said. "I clearly remember forgetting that."

On the recollections subject

Writing things down is the best secret of a good memory.

The true art of memory is the art of attention.

There's nothing we can do to improve ourselves so much as writing our memoirs.

Mark Twain said, "When I was younger I could remember anything whether it had happened or not."

If you don't think people have good memories, try repeating a joke you told them about a month ago.

One way to improve your memory is to lend people money.

These gems are from *Over the Hill & On a Roll* by Bob Phillips, a family, marriage, and child counselor, and the author of 72 books. In a section called "Sage Advice" he includes this quote by Henri Frederic Amiel:

"To know how to grow old is the masterwork of wisdom, and one of the most difficult chapters in the great art of living."

Sometimes prudence is a memory asset. Carol Channing occasionally asked audience members to pose questions during her nightclub acts. One evening a fellow asked, "Do you recall your most embarrassing moment?"

"Yes, I do," she said. "Next question."

Movie star Mae West had no problems with memory. "I used to be Snow White," she said, "but I drifted."

The elements of acceptance

An inscription on the ruins of a fifteenth-century cathedral in Amsterdam says, "It is so. It cannot be otherwise."

"As you and I march across the decades of time, we are going to meet a lot unpleasant situations that are so. They cannot be otherwise. We have our choice. We can either accept them as inevitable and adjust ourselves to them, or we can ruin our lives with rebellion and maybe end up with a nervous breakdown."

The observations above are those of Dale Carnegie in his book, *How to Stop Worrying and Start Living*. Does he advocate that we bow down to all adversities that come our way? "Not by a long shot," he declares. "That is mere fatalism. As long as there is a chance that we can save a situation, let's fight. But when common sense tells us that we are up against something that is so—and cannot be otherwise—then, in the name of our sanity, let's not 'look before and after and pine for what is not.'"

Columbia University's Dean Hawkes told Carnegie that one of his mottos was this Mother Goose rhyme:

For every ailment under the sun,
There is a remedy, or there is none;
If there be one, try to find it;
If there be none, never mind it.

Carnegie, as a young man, longed to become a Chautauqua lecturer. That fizzled, so he enrolled in the American Academy of Dramatic Arts in New York City, and landed a few roles. After he'd accepted the reality of a dead end on stage, a YMCA director okayed his proposal to conduct a public speaking course. In the first session, Carnegie ran out of material long before the announced conclusion. To fill the gap, he thought of a tactic: "You will now take turns standing before the group and talk about something that made you angry."

The technique helped the novices overcome their fear of speaking before a group, and gave Carnegie a method that made his subsequent courses successful. His books on public speaking were well received, but *How to Win Friends and Influence People* hit the best seller list. At the time of his death in 1955, it had sold five million copies in thirty-one languages.

'Age' is the acceptance of a term of years. But maturity is the glory of years.   —Martha Graham

Thoughts about departure time

Woody Allen said, "I don't want to achieve immortality through my work, I want to achieve it through not dying."

"Somebody should tell us, right at the start of our lives, that we are dying. Then we might live life to the limit, every minute of every day. Do it! I say. Whatever you want to do, do it now! There are only so many tomorrows."   — Pope Paul VI

I was a little taken aback when I got my receipt from the funeral parlor, on the bottom of the receipt, after the bill, it read, "Thank you. Please come again."

If you spend all your time worrying about dying, living isn't going to be much fun. (From the television show Roseanne.)

In Roger Rosenblatt's book, *Rules for Aging,* he titles one brief section "Abjure fame but avoid obscurity." (The dictionary defines abjure as "To recant solemnly; repudiate.") He comments about the perils of pursuing fame. "If instead . . . you are more interested in simply meriting the approval of peers, the chances are better that you will accomplish this by drawing attention to the things you do rather than to some shimmering persona that you have manufactured for public inspection."

He describes Lewis Thomas a good example of this notion. When Thomas, the author of *The Lives of a Cell* and a biologist-physician-philosopher as well, was ill with lymphoma, Rosenblatt, his friend for many years, asked if he could interview him. "I told him that he had helped so many people understand the nature of living that it would be valuable if he could also tell them something of dying."

They talked for the next two years, but Thomas decided "It was more important to know how to live than how to die." He said the best criterion for life was to determine whether it has been of use to others. "If it were useful, it would be noticed."

Rosenblatt's article appeared in the *New York Times* magazine ten days before Thomas died in 1993. "During those ten days, the magazine and I received hundreds of letters from Lewis's readers over the years who wanted to thank him for the learning and the wisdom his writing had giving them."

Bobby was with his grandfather and posed a question: "Grandpa, do you know how to make animal sounds?"

"I sure do," he said. "What sort of animal sound would you like to hear?"

"How about a toad? Do you know how to sound like a toad?"

"Sure," said the grandfather, cupping his hand to his mouth. "Croaaak croaaak. How did you like that?"

"Yipee!" Bobby yelled, jumping up and down, "We're going to Miami!"

"Huh? Why's that?"

"Because Grandma said so," Bobby replied. "She said that after you croak we'll all go to Miami!"

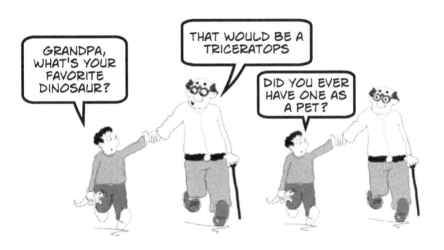

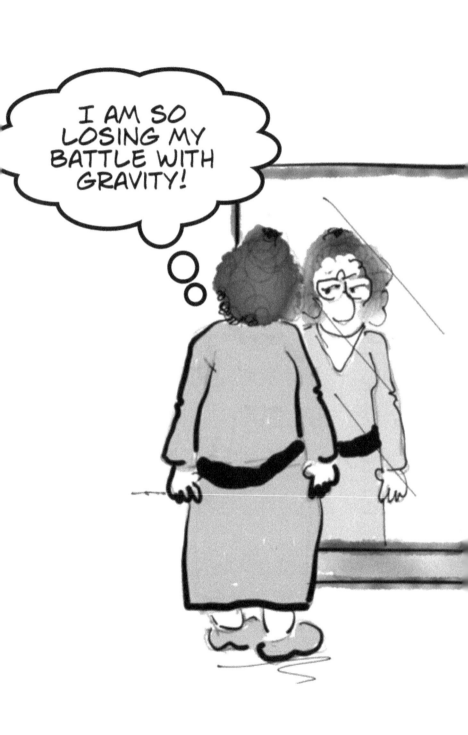

Working out, or possibly in

Some of the commentary about exercise deals with reasons why people can't or won't do it:

If God had wanted me to touch my toes, he would have put them on my knees.
If you want to take up cross-country skiing, start with a small country.
The trouble with jogging is that, by the time you realize you're not in shape for it, its too far to walk back. — Franklin P. Jones
I like long walks, especially when they're taken by people who annoy me.— Fred Allen
The only reason I would take up jogging is so I could hear heavy breathing again.   — Erma Bombeck

"Exercise is the best anti-aging medicine," says Dr. Sanjay Gupta. It helps manage weight, improves muscle and bone strength, and even lifts your spirits. It can also add years to your life.

"People have been looking for the secret to a long and healthy life for millennia," said Neil Resnick, MD, chief of the division of geriatrics and director of the University of Pittsburgh Institute on Aging. "It turns out the most powerful intervention is exercise."

A study at Harvard found that exercise can be at least as effective as prescription drugs when it comes to preventing common conditions such as heart disease, stroke, and diabetes. As Dr. Resnick points out, a little exercise can go a long way. One study found that just 15 minutes a day of moderate-intensity activity extended people's lives by three years. "Exercising at very light levels reduced deaths from any cause by 14 percent."

"It doesn't require being an Olympic athlete to get these

health benefits," said Resnick. "You don't have to go to a gym and break a huge sweat. You don't have to lift massive amounts of weight. You don't have to run a marathon. If you walk 30 minutes a day, five days a week, you're getting that benefit."

Researchers from the University College London found that "healthy agers," or physically active older adults, had a lower risk for chronic diseases such as arthritis. Evidence suggests that exercise also helps delay cognitive impairment. "We're probably sort of genetically wired for physical activity," said William Hall, MD, at the University of Rochester's School of Medicine. "People who exercise tend to have better immune systems, and the body doesn't suffer from inflammation as much."

In a remote mountain area of southern Russia, a land known as Abkhasia, people don't concern themselves with exercise. They don't need to. Many reputedly achieve life spans of 100-plus because they spend most of their adult lives working in tea fields in temperatures usually between 50 and 55 degrees. Even after retirement they remain active gardening and walking. Their diet is a plus factor. Meals consist mainly of home-grown vegetables and dairy products, including yogurt, with moderate amounts of grains, nuts, and meat.

As for the rest of us in the West, most of us lose muscle mass as we age and it's replaced with fat. "At 65, almost half the body weight of both men and women is fat, double what it was in their twenties," says Deepak Chopra, MD, in his book *Ageless Body, Timeless Mind.*

Then there are the skeptics like Ellen DeGeneres, who says, "I really don't think I need buns of steel. I'd be happier with buns of cinnamon."

Idealism moves you

It can be both fun and satisfying to help others. When Robert Fulghum served as a Unitarian minister, he found the Salvation Army at work wherever human need was greatest. Members of his church "kept the kettles boiling for the Salvation Army every December," he said in his book *Uh-Oh*.

His son, Sam, would ring the brass bell with ferocious insistence, point to the black kettle, and shout, "IN THE POT. PLEASE PUT SOMETHING IN THE POT FOR THE BABY JEEZIS!" Next he sang "Jingle Bells" in his sincere little voice, and oftentimes people filled the pot to the brim.

On the road home, he would inquire nonstop, "If there is a Salvation Army, is there a Salvation Navy?" and "Do they have tanks?" plus "Are angels the Salvation Air Force?"

The church members once formed a band for the purpose of persuading donors to give generously. Fulghum realized a dream by playing the bass drum. Sam clanged his bell and shouted, "HELP, HELP THE POOR CHILDREN." The music sounded a bit Brazilian, Fulghum admitted, but, "We raised so much money the kettle was filled to overflowing."

The Salvation Army switched to hiring the unemployed to seek Christmastime gifts. So Fulghum decided it was easier to send a check in the mail, which he did.

Then he had change of heart and said, "It does no good-solves nothing-to distance myself from the front lines of human need by using the mail as a safe shelter. I believe that serving the best ends of humanity means getting out in the middle of it just as it is, not staying home writing checks and thinking hopeful thoughts.

"The world does not need tourists who ride by in a bus clucking their tongues. The world as it is needs those who will love it enough to change it, with what they have, where they are.

"And you're damned right that's idealistic. No apology. When idealism goes into the trash as junk mail, we're finished."

When life takes a turn

I love being married. It's so great to find the one special person you want to annoy for the rest of your life.   — Rita Rudner

A couple is lying in bed. The man says, "I am going to make you the happiest woman in the world." The woman replies, "I'll miss you . . ."

We joke about matrimonial matters, but there are grim times for many women because they end up without a mate toward the end of their lives. The life expectancy for women is nearly eight years longer than for men.

"Widowhood is a rite of passage in the strongest sense of the word," says Frances Weaver in her book, *The Girls with the Grandmother Faces*. "Our lives have changed and can never be the same again. The friends, the social life, the financial priorities, our relationships with our children, daily routines and leisure time, the way we eat, the way we sleep are all new. It's almost like starting over."

Her husband died when they were both 55. She admits to some mistakes afterward, such as buying a condo near family and friends, only to discover that "I wanted to make myself the center of everyone's lives, although I would have knocked anyone out of the ballpark for suggesting this as my motive."

Weaver offers a list of don'ts, including don't drop in unannounced or insist on family gatherings for all of the holidays. She decided at the age of 75 to move into a retirement community and take advantage of the care, companionship and security.

"Making choices implies an acceptance of risk . . .but risk pays off in new adventure, friends and excitement," she states.

"It often leads to greater discoveries of our own capabilities."

One woman in a grief support group said that she and her late husband made a living trust. "When he died there were no money problems."

There can be laughter to lessen the grief. For example, the cartoon of three men with hair wildly askew in a funeral parlor office. The one on the telephone is saying, "I realize we all grieve in our own way, ma'am, but the staff did not appreciate the fireworks you put in your late husband's pockets."

Then there's the fellow whose tombstone reads, "Now I know something you don't."

Declare your purpose

Lawrence Peter Berra, best know as Yogi Berra, died on September 22, 2015. He achieved distinction during his major league baseball years, but became even better known for his sayings that appealed to many who didn't follow the sport. Here are some examples:

If the world were perfect, it wouldn't be.
Take it with a grin of salt.
You can observe a lot by just watching.
It ain't over til it's over.

Always go to other people's funerals, otherwise they won't come to yours.

If you don't know where you're going, you might end up someplace else.

Several of Yogi's quotations present a good lead-in to some provocative questions posed in Jim Loehr's book *The Power of Story*. His main one is this: have you determined the purpose of your life?

"Once you find your purpose, you have a chance to live a story that moves you and those around you," he says.

That purpose, he continues, might be to leave the world a better place, to honor God, to live to one hundred, or to seek out adventure and risk. To help his readers compose their statements, he lists these questions:

How do you want to be remembered?
What is the legacy you most want to leave to others?

How would you most like people to eulogize you at your funeral?

What is worth dying for?

What makes your life really worth living?

In what areas of your life must you truly be extraordinary to fulfill your destiny?

Jim Loehr wants you to establish your ultimate mission. "By envisioning the end of your life, you are . . .pausing to define what could reasonably be called a purposeful life, as lived by you," he declares. He suggests envisioning your tombstone and the word or words below the name, date of birth, and date of death. It makes you think about where you're headed.

Here are a few tombstone messages that may not exactly fit his guideline:

"I am ready to meet my Maker. Whether my Maker is prepared for the great ordeal of meeting me is another matter."
— Winston Churchill

"The best is yet to come."   — Frank Sinatra

"That's all, folks!"   — Mel Blanc

"Here lies/Johnny Yeast. /Pardon me/For not rising."
-In Ruidoso, New Mexico

"Here lies an honest lawyer/And that is Strange."
-Sir John Strange, an English attorney

Aging while getting better

Goodman Ace, a writer whose columns appeared in the *Saturday Review*, said that birthdays went out of style at his house when his wife asked, "Well, dear, how do you feel this morning on your birthday?"

"Old," he answered.

She scolded him, then said, "Don't say you're old, just say you're getting older."

After he complied, she asked, "Now, don't you feel better?"

And thus began years of not mentioning or celebrating birthdays. However, on the days following the birthdays, a gift invariably turned up on the breakfast table or a night stand. Most of the time it was a sweater for him and perfume for her.

"And you want to know something?" Ace said. "It has taken years off my age."

His wife, Jane, didn't mention his latest birthday, but made an oblique reference. "I heard a funny joke today about age," she said. "A man is as old as he looks. A woman is as old as she likes. Ha, ha, ha."

"You heard that today?" he asked.

"Yes, don't you get it, dear?"

"That joke is not old. It's only getting older."

You need to maintain your sense of humor and deflect anger, according to Dr. Walter M. Bortz. In his book, *We Live Too Short and Die Too Long*, he says, "Make each day an opportunity for optimism for yourself and others. If you're thinking positively, it creates the expectation that something good is going to happen," he adds. It also opens the door to new options for success.

While we're on this topic of aging, consider this observation by Daniel J. Metzger: "You're only as old as you feel—the next day." As for the final phase: "Death is a very dull, dreary affair, and my advice to you is to have nothing whatsoever to do with it," maintains Somerset Maugham.

(These two gems are from *The Official Explanations* compiled by Paul Dickson.)

What you say in your memoir

So you're thinking about writing your life story. You might have some fun with it, somewhat like the authors of the following:

Everything Is Perfect When You're a Liar by Kelly Oxford
Let's Pretend This Never Happened by Jenny Lawson
Hyperbole and a Half by Allie Brosh
Can't We Talk About Something More Pleasant? by Roy Chart
People Are Unappealing: Even Me by Sara Barron
I Remember Nothing by Nora Ephron
Dead End Gene Pool by Wendy Burden

William Zinsser's book about memoir writing is called *Inventing the Truth.* It's an apt title, he declares, because "It states the most important principle for writing the story of your life: mere facts aren't enough. No matter how many details you diligently collect about the people and places and events in your past, they won't add up to a memoir. You must make a narrative arrangement."

Make it compelling, he continues, by using the storyteller's rule of maintaining tension and momentum. "You are the central actor in your story, and you must give yourself a plot," and it's okay to rearrange and compress the story to give it dramatic shape, he says.

Some people might benefit from this advice by England's Rev. Sydney Smith: "In composing, as a general rule, run your pen through every other word you have written; you have no idea what vigor it will give your style."

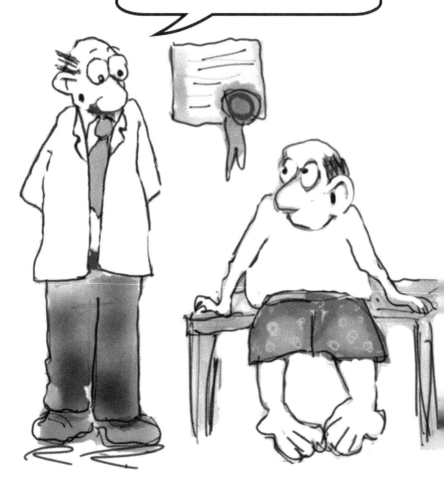

Is laughter a good medicine?

Colonoscopies are important medical procedures that have saved lives. And yet they're as popular as, well, a colonoscopy. Here are comments purportedly made by patients to physicians during their procedures:

"Now I know how a Muppet feels!"

"Could you write a note for my wife saying that my head is not up there?"

"Any sign of the trapped miners, chief?"
Source: Dave Barry, in the *Miami Herald*

The physiological study of laughter has its own name: "gelotology." Research has shown that laughing is more than just a person's voice and movement, according to *Neuroscience for Kids*. Laughter requires the coordination of many muscles, and also:

Increases blood pressure
Increases heart rate
Changes breathing
Reduces levels of certain neurochemicals (catecholamines, hormones)
Provides a boost to the immune system

Can laughter improve health? It may help people relax because muscle tension is reduced after laughing. A good deep laugh helps people with respiratory problems by clearing mucus and aiding ventilation. Perhaps laughing can also aid cardiac patients by giving the heart a bit of a workout. Some hospital

"Humor Rooms," "Comedy Carts," and clowns may speed a patient's recovery and boost morale.

However, in a few cases, laughing has caused a heart attack or a stroke. Also, after abdominal surgery, people should not laugh too hard because they could tear out their stitches accidentally. Care should also be used in patients with broken ribs. So, try not to be too funny around these people.

A Vanderbilt University study estimated that just 10-15 minutes of laughter a day can burn up to 40 calories. Meanwhile, a University of Maryland study found that a sense of humor can protect against heart disease.

Lower cortisol? Lower stress? Sounds pretty good. But researchers insist the benefits are even greater. "There are several benefits to humor and laughter," explained Gurinder S. Bains, a Ph.D. candidate at Loma Linda University, who co-authored the study. "Older adults need to have a better quality of life. Incorporating time to laugh, through social interaction with friends, enjoying exercise in a group setting, or even watching 20 minutes of humor on TV daily, can enhance your learning ability and delayed recall."

The results are intriguing, but don't be too hasty in ditching that treadmill. One piece of chocolate has about 50 calories; at the rate of 50 calories per hour, losing one pound would require about 12 hours of concentrated laughter!

Something we need to jog

Your marriage is in trouble if your wife says, "You're only interested in one thing," and you can't remember what it is.
— Milton Berle

Happiness is nothing more than good health and a bad memory.   — Albert Schweitzer

Right now I'm having amnesia and deja vu at the same time-I think I've forgotten this before.   — Steven Wright

One tip that Betty Fielding suggests for remembering names of people you've just met is to form a mental image that includes the person, the place, and the context. In her book, *The Memory Manual,* she adds that you can also imagine the person's name on a name tag as you tune in to what is said, how it's said, and the mannerisms that accompany the words. She includes this example:

"In recalling a man you met in a clubhouse setting, you might think: I can see us standing in front of the fireplace and wondering where the manager got such fine big logs. Now what was his name? Oh, yes, it was Dave Perez."

Her book provides ten things seniors can do to improve their memory. They range from understanding how memory works, focusing, organizing, dealing with stress, and becoming your own mentor.

I constantly walk into a room and I don't remember why; but for some reason, I think there's going to be a clue in the fridge.
— Caroline Rhea

Marriage is the alliance of two people, one of whom never remembers birthdays and the other never forgets them.

— Ogden Nash

There are three signs of old age: one is memory loss . . . I can't remember the other four.   — Christopher Stevens

Don't ignore the basics

In his 1841 inaugural address, President William Henry Harrison spoke for nearly one hour and forty minutes. Cold winds buffeted the March 4 event, held on the Capitol's east portico. Despite the stormy weather, he declined to wear a coat or a hat. He caught a cold that developed into pneumonia, and died a month later.

He should have known better, according to *Presidential Trivia* by Richard Lederer. Harrison had studied medicine for a year at the University of Pennsylvania.

Colds, unfortunately, are incurable. You treat the symptoms. So it makes sense to prevent them. The basics include ample sleep, healthy diet, and exercise. Wash your hands frequently and keep them away from your head. People touch their faces 3.6 times per hour and touch common objects such as tables, phones, and doorknobs 3.3 times per hour. This is one of the most common ways germs can be transmitted from person to person.

Grandparents love nothing more in this world than their grandchildren. Unfortunately, with kids come germs, and all those hugs and kisses can transmit germs to an older adult.

Avoid touching your eyes, nose or mouth as much as possible to prevent germs from being transmitted to those locations.

Sometimes, it is a good thing to be a little anti-social during cold and flu season. Keeping distance between yourself and people who are ill is a good step in avoiding a cold. Elderly individuals should consider keeping their distance in cars and elevators or in areas where large groups of people congregate, such as malls.

According to the American Lung Association, all adults over the age of fifty need to get a seasonal flu shot.

It was autumn, and Indians on their remote reservation asked the chief if the winter was going to be cold or mild. He was a new chief, and had never been taught the old secrets. When he looked at the sky, he couldn't tell what the weather was going to be.

He told his tribe that the winter was indeed going to be cold and they should collect wood to be prepared. After several days he got an idea. He went to the phone booth, called the National Weather Service and asked, "Is the coming winter going to be cold?"

"It looks like this winter is going to be quite cold indeed," the meteorologist responded.

So the chief went back to his people and told them to collect even more wood in order to be prepared. A week later he called the weather service again.

"Is it going to be a very cold winter?"

"Yes," the man replied, "it's going to be very cold."

The chief went back to his people and ordered them to collect every scrap of wood they could find. Two weeks later he called again. "Are you absolutely sure that the winter is going to be very cold?"

"Absolutely," the man said. "It's going to be one of the coldest winters ever."

"How can you be so sure?" the chief asked.

The weatherman replied, "The Indians are collecting wood like crazy."

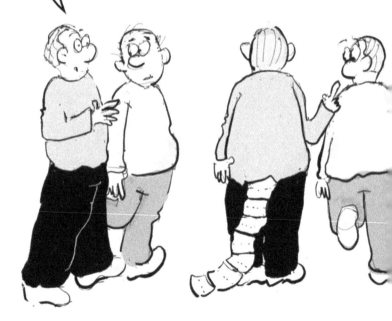

Traveling tips and troubles

A woman from the country was visiting the big city for the first time. She checked in at the hotel and let the porter take her bags. She followed him in. But as the door closed, her face fell. "Young man," she said to him. "I may be old, but I'm not retarded. I paid a lot of money for this room, but it's nothing like I expected. It's too small and there's no air conditioning. There's not even a bed here!"

Porter replied: "This isn't your room. This is the lift."

Yes, things can go awry when you're traveling. Peg Bracken dealt with many of the challenges in her book, *But I Wouldn't Have Missed It for the World*. Take, for example, decisions on which clothes to take.

"What you pack is a compromise, as a rule, between how you want to look and what you want to bother with, just as a woman's figure is generally a compromise between how she wants to look and what she wants to eat," Bracken writes.

Don't take brand new, untried clothes, she advises. Pretest everything. Take old, dependable clothes and you'll have a good excuse to buy something new when you get there.

Another crucial item to take along: a candy bar. "In any long or longish journey, there is usually one critical moment when the traveler finds himself starving to death, owing to factors beyond his control, like no food in sight," Bracken says in a work that, even though it was published in 1973, still contains good tips for today.

She favors the use of a travel agent. "Doing your own complicated trip—like your own brain surgery—will nearly always result in a mussier, more expensive, and more painful experience than you had planned on."

Here in the U.S., cut hotel expenses by avoiding the coffee shop for breakfast "and room service for everything," she advises. "Cookies, dried fruit, instant coffee, and an immersion heater all travel well in your suitcase. So do wine or whiskey when properly swaddled."

"When you come to a fork in the road . . . take it."
—Yogi Berra

"Kilometers are shorter than miles. Save gas, take your next trip in kilometers."   — George Carlin

"If you've seen one redwood tree, you've seen them all."
— Ronald Reagan

"Too often travel, instead of broadening the mind, merely lengthens the conversations."   — Elizabeth Drew

"Another well-known Paris landmark is the Arc de Triomphe, a moving monument to the many brave women and men who have died trying to visit it."   — Dave Barry

"Thanks to the interstate highway system, it is now possible to travel from coast to coast without seeing anything."
— Charles Kuralt

"The worst thing about being a tourist is having other tourists recognize you as a tourist."   — Russell Baker

"You can find your way across this country using burger joints the way a navigator uses stars."   — Charles Kuralt

"You got to be careful if you don't know where you're going, because you might not get there."   — Yogi Berra

Something to count on

Shop signs

Outside a dress shop, Hong Kong:

> LADIES HAVE FITS UPSTAIRS.

Tailor shop, Greece:

> ORDER YOUR SUMMERS SUIT. BECAUSE IS BIG RUSH,
> WE WILL EXECUTE CUSTOMERS IN STRICT ROTATION.

On the door of a Moscow hotel room:

> IF THIS IS YOUR FIRST VISIT TO THE USSR,
> YOU ARE WELCOME TO IT.

England plumber's van

> THE LONE DRAINER-HE COME PRONTO

The late *San Francisco Chronicle* columnist Charles McCabe once wrote, "When the world gets too much with me, there will intrude on my morbid meditations a cautionary voice. It says: 'No matter how bad things are, no matter they weigh upon you, there is no man so bereft that he cannot find things to love, if only he can and will.'"

Some of us, he says, love our disabilities. "Feeling sorry for yourself is the cheapest of luxuries," he adds. When it happens, he counts his blessings even though it may be uphill work. His list of things for which he was grateful included four great kids, and a "much-abused, but seemingly intact liver." Also, "I haven't gone sour on life, or most of the people who live it."

He enjoyed reading, travel, music, and "I like women, especially women with strong appetites."

McCabe died in 1983.

Becky was 73 and just got her first computer. After her son spent over two hours teaching her how to use it, she was sure she knew everything there was to know about computers.

Unfortunately, one day she couldn't get it to start so she called an IT guy to come take a look at it. He managed to fix the issue in a few minutes and started to leave.

She overheard the IT guy on the phone with his boss telling him about the issue, and was certain she'd taken care of it the right way. "Excuse me, if you don't mind me asking," Becky said to the man. "I couldn't help overhearing you on the phone. What exactly is an Id ten T problem? Just so I can tell my son." The man smiled, took out a pen, and explained, "It stands for this: I-D-1-0-T."

Tapping into the power

Richard Carter's book, *The Golden Years Are a Crock*, melds humor with some grim facts of life. For example, nearly half of the people over the age of 85 experience some form of dementia. Carter would say this means you can keep repeating the same joke to a lot of people.

It isn't funny, though, if seniors can't write checks to pay their bills. Also, if they didn't inform their doctors to not take heroic measures when their time was up, they may face tragic consequences.

The best way to avoid calamities such as these? Arrange for a power of attorney. This legal document enables the person or agency that you select to act on your behalf if you are incapacitated or unable to make decisions.

In the case of illness, you can have a durable power of attorney for medical care. If you empower someone you trust as your durable power of attorney for finances, that person or agency can manage your investments, pay your bills, and handle other money matters if you can't do so. By obtaining these documents, you may one day help your loved ones avoid feeling their lives are a crock because of court proceedings or hospital travail.

One gauge of the well-being of seniors, according to Richard Carter: "For those over 70, if they can get up at night, find the bathroom, and remember how to get back to bed, they are in excellent health."

"Forgetfulness is the beginning of happiness as fear is the beginning of wisdom."   — Gabriel de Tarde

SENILITY PRAYER

God grant me the senility
to forget the people
I never liked anyway,
the good fortune
to run into the ones I do,
and the eyesight to tell the difference.

Peter Mitchell received the Nobel Prize in Chemistry (1978) for his contribution to the understanding of biological energy transfer through the formulation of the chemiosmotic theory. Some ten years after the divorce from his first wife, Eileen, Mitchell attended the wedding of their daughter, and he noticed a woman who looked familiar. He asked whether he knew her, and she replied "Yes, I was your first wife."

Mitchell was keenly aware of his forgetfulness; he even coined the expression "forgetory," which is the opposite of memory.

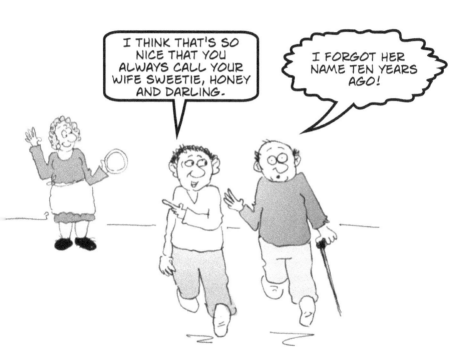

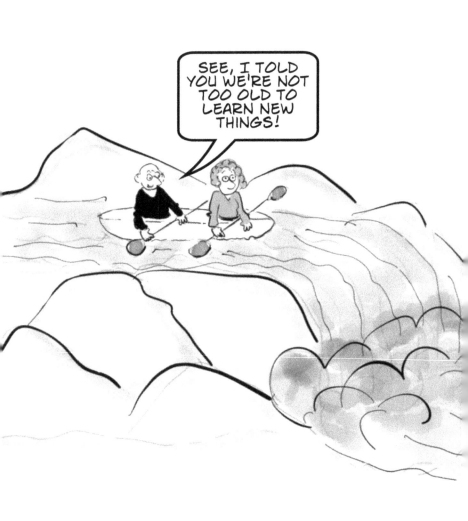

Win some, lose some

Everyone should prepare for life's conclusion, and Guy Browning provides a couple of interesting tips for that occasion. "Include a few surprises in your will," he says. "Leave a pair of your underpants to your lawyers. Leave something valuable that you don't actually own to that greedy person so he or she can spend a lifetime looking for it."

"Just because you're dying doesn't mean you can't have fun," he declares in his book, *Never Hit a Jellyfish with a Spade*.

Judith Viorst's book *Necessary Losses* includes cogent thoughts about growing older and the losses that take place along the way. "Old age can be active or disengaged, feisty or serene, a keeping up of our front or a dropping of masks, a consolidation of what we know and what we've done before, or a new—even unconventional—exploration," she says. At which point, she prints the poem by Jenny Joseph entitled "Warning":

When I am an old woman I shall wear purple
With a red hat which doesn't go, and doesn't suit me,
And I shall spend my pension on brandy and summer gloves
And satin sandals, and say we've no money for butter.
I shall sit down on the pavement when I'm tired
And gobble up samples in shops and press alarm bells
And run my stick along the public railings
And make up for the sobriety of my youth.
I shall go out in my slippers in the rain
And pick the flowers in other people's gardens
And learn to spit.

Viorst then observes: "Less rebellious old ladies may prefer to rock in their rocking chairs. That too, of course, can make for a good old age." She provides ideas about coping with losses during infancy, childhood, adulthood, marriage, and the final years. "We may find that a good old age demands a capacity for what is called 'ego transcendence,'" she says. It includes:

"A capacity to feel pleasure in the pleasures of other people.

"A capacity for concern about events not directly related to our self-interest.

"A capacity to invest ourselves (though we won't be around to see it) in tomorrow's world."

By bestowing some form of legacy to the next generation we can constructively deal with the grief we feel over the loss of ourselves, she maintains.

And Guy Browning's view? "Death can be as simple as falling off a log. Which is why you should steer clear of logs."

Take some time for this

You can't turn back the clock. But you can wind it up again.
— Bonnie Prudden

A day wasted on others is not wasted on one's self.
— Charles Dickens

Time is money, especially when you are talking to a lawyer
or buying a commercial.   — Frank Dane

To live is so startling it leaves little time for anything else.
— Emily Dickinson

Without music to decorate it, time is just a bunch of boring
production deadlines or dates by which bills must be paid.
— Frank Zappa

No man goes before his time - unless the boss leaves early.
— Groucho Marx

There's never enough time to do it right, but there's always
enough time to do it over.   — Jack Bergman

We must use time as a tool, not as a couch.
— John F. Kennedy

People who cannot find time for recreation are obliged
sooner or later to find time for illness.   — John Wanamaker

I am definitely going to take a course on time management...
just as soon as I can work it into my schedule. — Louis E. Boone

Time is a great healer, but a poor beautician.
— Lucille S. Harper

There is more to life than increasing its speed.
— Mahatma Gandhi

The bad news is time flies. The good news is you're the pilot.
— Michael Altshuler

So you'd like to manage your time better. Try these tech-
niques recommended by Denis Waitley in *Being the Best*:

Use a self-development plan. Write down the knowledge you
require, the behavior plans you are changing, and the improve-
ments you desire. Star items you achieve and add others to the
list.

Begin each day with a question. What will you accomplish
today? What will lead you closer to your purpose?

Learn from good role models. Talk to people who do well at
what you want to do most. Learn everything you can from them.

The trouble with being punctual is no one is there to appreciate it.

You can boost the brain

An alien walked into a shop and told the owner that he came from Mars and wanted to buy a brain for research. "How much is this one?" he asked.

"That one is a monkey brain, and it's $20," the owner said.

"How much is that one?" the alien asked.

"That one is a female brain, and it's $100," the owner replied.

"And how much is that one?" the alien asked.

"That one is a male's brain and it is $500," the owner said.

"Why so expensive?" the alien asked.

The owner answered, "Well, it's hardly been used."

You can lower your risk of cognitive decline with the same habits that are also good for your health in general, says Angela Timashenka Geiger. The Alzheimer's Association's chief strategy officer suggests these steps:

1. Engage in regular cardiovascular exercise that elevates your heart rate and increases blood flow to the brain and body.

2. Take a class at a college or community center or online. Formal education in any stage of life will help reduce your risk of cognitive decline and dementia.

3. Obesity, high blood pressure, and diabetes negatively impact cognitive health. Take care of your heart, and your brain just might follow.

4. Avoid head injuries.

5. Stay socially engaged. Find ways to be part of your local community or simply share activities with friends and family.

6. Get enough sleep. Take care of conditions like insomnia or sleep apnea that may result in problems with memory and thinking.

7. Seek medical treatment if you have symptoms of depression, anxiety, or other mental health concerns. Also, try to manage stress.

8. Pursue social activities that are meaningful to you. Or simply share activities with friends and family.

9. Challenge yourself to think in new ways. Complete a jigsaw puzzle, do something artistic, or build a piece of furniture. Play games, such as bridge, that make you think strategically.

Geiger says research suggests that combining good nutrition with mental, social, and physical activities may have a greater benefit in maintaining or improving brain health than any single activity.

Why can't you trust an atom?
Because they make up everything.

With age comes wisdom

Robert Orben once said, "Time flies. It's up to you to be the navigator."

Wisdom consists of "making the best use of available knowledge," according to one definition. Dr. Gene D. Cohen says that isn't completely satisfying. "For most people, wisdom also connotes a perspective that supports the long-term common good over the short-term good for an individual," he says.

When faced with a decision, you'll take into account the results of previous choices you've made or ones you know about. They help you anticipate what may come next. Your wise choices also may hinge on your intuition, reason, and spirit, Dr. Cohen says. "It is fundamentally the manifestation of developmental intelligence—a mature integration of thinking skills, emotional intelligence, judgment, social skills and life experience."

As people age, they tend to sever superficial or unsatisfying relationships. Thus they can spend their time with people they care about and feel comfortable with.

The funny wisdoms of life:

Never miss an opportunity to make others happy, even if you have to leave them alone in order to do it.
— Author unknown

I refuse to answer that question on the grounds that I don't know the answer.   — Douglas Adams

The empty vessel makes the greatest sound.
—William Shakespeare

Silence and smile are two powerful words. Smile is the way to solve many problems and silence is the way to avoid many problems.   — Anon

Knowledge talks, wisdom listens.

There cannot be a crisis next week. My schedule is already full.   —Henry Kissinger

He has all the virtues I dislike, and none of the vices I admire.   — Winston Churchill

I used to be indecisive, now I'm not so sure.   —W.C. Fields

In the book of life, the answers aren't in the back.   — Charlie Brown

To succeed in life, you need three things: a wishbone, a backbone, and a funny bone.   — Reba McEntire

Mistakes are painful when they happen, but years later a collection of mistakes called *Experience* leads us to success.

Everyone's going nutty

A guy goes into a bar. He's sitting on the stool, enjoying his drink when he hears, "You look great!" He looks around-there's nobody near him. He hears the voice again, "No, really, you look terrific."

The guy looks around again. Nobody. He hears, "Is that a new shirt or something? Because you are absolutely glowing!" He then realizes that the voice is coming from a dish of nuts on the bar.

"Hey," the guy calls to the bartender, "What's with the nuts?"

"Oh," the bartender answers, "They're complimentary."

As it turns out, nuts are also healthy. The Dr. Dean Ornish's Program for Reversing Heart Disease now allows a limited amount of nuts and seeds, based on research showing they improve cardiovascular health and reduce diseases such as type 2 diabetes. The inclusion of nuts and seeds does not change the daily percentage of calories from fat, it just provides more choices.

For example, one serving could include 5 almonds, 9 pistachios, 1 whole walnut, 3 pecan halves, 2 cashews, 6 peanuts, 5 tsp. ground flax seeds, 2 tsp. shelled chia or sunflower seeds, and 5 tsp. pumpkin seeds.

A five-year randomized control study of 7,216 patients, who were all at high risk of heart disease, revealed the group that included nuts cut their incidence of strokes in half. The results also showed increased nut consumption reduced risk of mortality.

There's a great metaphor that one of my doctors uses: if a fish is swimming in a dirty tank and it gets sick, do you take it to the vet and amputate the fin? No, you clean the water. So, I cleaned up my system. By eating organic raw greens, nuts and healthy fats, I am flooding my body with enzymes, vitamins and oxygen.

—Kris Carr

"I hate television. I hate it as much as peanuts. But I can't stop eating peanuts.   —Orson Welles

A bargain-priced remedy

Josh phoned his heart surgeon to schedule an appointment for an immediate surgery.

"I'm sorry," the receptionist answered, "we don't have anything available for the next three weeks."

"But I could die by then!"

"No problem, just call before to cancel the appointment."

The medical profession would like to cancel or at least lessen heart attacks. One in four deaths in the United States every year results from heart problems. The number of people diagnosed with heart failure is expected to increase from about 5.7 million today to nearly 8 million by 2030, according to the American Heart Association.

"There's been a huge effort and so much focus on heart failure," said University of Pennsylvania cardiologist Mariell Jessup, M.D. "But heart failure, for all intents and purposes, is a problem with the elderly, and the elderly population has increased."

All of us should watch for these warning signs and symptoms:

Chest pain or discomfort.
Upper body pain or discomfort in the arms, back, neck, jaw, or upper stomach.
Shortness of breath.
Nausea, lightheadedness, or cold sweats.

A Harvard Medical School study of 22,000 male physicians found that in four-and-a-half-years one-half of the group that took one aspirin every other day suffered 139 heart attacks and ten heart attack deaths. The other half who took placebos had 239 heart attacks and 26 heart attack deaths.

People over 50, after discussing it with their doctors, can lessen the risk by taking one adult aspirin every other day, according to *Smart Ways to Stay Young and Healthy* by Bradley Gascoigne, M.D., and Julie Irwin. They add that adults who have had one heart attack can lower their odds of a second one with low-dose aspirin every other day.

In another study, the American Cancer Society found that aspirin use reduced the rate of colon cancer by 40 percent.

About ten percent of people with severe asthma are also allergic to aspirin— and, in fact, to all products containing salicylic acid, aspirin's key ingredient, including some cold medications, fruits, and food seasonings and additives. That percentage skyrockets to 30 to 40 percent for older asthmatics who also suffer from sinusitis or nasal polyps.

Acute sensitivity to aspirin is also seen in a small percentage of the general population without asthma—particularly people with ulcers and other bleeding conditions. Always consult your doctor before using any medication, and do not apply aspirin externally if you are allergic to taking it internally.

—Reader's Digest

When I get a headache I take two aspirins and keep away from children, just like it says on the bottle.

Lots have bones to pick

Joan Rivers said, "My bones click so much that dolphins try to pick up on me."

Her osteoporosis condition was no laughing matter, but she made light of it— and made progress.

At the age of 64, Joan discovered it was stalking her, waiting for an opportunity to make a wisecrack of its own: snap, crackle, pop. She developed these one-liners about ways to discourage osteoporosis:

Walk everywhere
Choose the stairs over the elevator
Exercise three times a week with weights
Take nutritional supplements

This regimen strengthened her bones, and her stage presence. Joan became an ambassador for the National Osteoporosis Foundation and championed reversing the symptoms of the disease. She said that while people look beautiful on the outside, they should pay more attention to keeping their bones strong. After all, beauty is bone deep.

Joan Rivers, described as the Queen of comedy in America, and author of twelve best-selling books, died on September 4, 2014, of cardiac arrest during an operation on her vocal cords.

The National Osteoporosis Foundation estimates that 10.2 million adults have osteoporosis and another 43.4 million have low bone mass. Its study projects that by 2030, the number of adults over age 50 with osteoporosis or low bone mass will grow to 71.2 million (a 29% increase from 2010).

What can you do to protect your bones? Get enough calcium

and vitamin D by eating yogurt, cheese, milk, sardines with bones, and green, leafy vegetables. Engage in regular exercise. Avoid smoking and limit alcohol to one drink per day for women and two per day for men.

Here are a few of Joan Rivers' candid comments:

People say that money is not the key to happiness, but I always figured if you have enough money, you can have a key made.

I was born in 1962 ... and the room next to me was 1963.

My best birth control now is just to leave the lights on.

I blame my mother for my poor sex life. All she told me was, "The man goes on top and the woman underneath." For three years my husband and I slept in bunk beds.

I've had so much plastic surgery, when I die, they will donate my body to Tupperware.

Not all plastic surgeons are good. My cousin went to one and told him she wanted to turn back the hands of time. Now she has a face that could stop a clock.

I was so ugly that they sent my picture to Ripley's Believe It or Not. He sent it back and said, "I don't believe it."

Fighting the isolation urge

The worst loneliness is to not be comfortable with yourself.
—Mark Twain

You cannot be lonely if you like the person you're alone with.
—Wayne Dyer

I never feel lonely if I've got a book—they're like old friends. Even if you're not reading them over and over again, you know they are there. And they're part of your history. They sort of tell a story about your journey through life.   —Emilia Fox

Life is too short to waste on suffering from core loneliness, according to psychotherapist Ross A. Rosenberg. He recommends that you open up, take a chance and access the hidden part of you that deserves true and loving companions. Heal your childhood wounds. Learn to love yourself and eliminate loneliness from your life. His suggestions include:

Catch your inner critic's thoughts like "I am too fat for anybody to want to date." Replace negative self-talk with affirming messages. Fight the urge to isolate. Weed out the toxic relationships and create space in your life for relationships that fuel your spirit.

Even if there is only one person to start with, nurture your support network, then expand it. Open yourself up, take risks, and allow yourself to be vulnerable. Tell people what you need from them to alleviate the loneliness. Don't wait for an invitation. Be willing to take a risk, be proactive, and invite people to share in your life, whether it is for coffee, lunch, a walk, an event, or a gathering in your home.

Recognize the importance of being alone, enjoying solitude and connecting with your deeper self. Consider therapy. It can change your thinking and relationship patterns and help you achieve the life you want.

If you learn to really sit with loneliness and embrace it for the gift that it is . . . an opportunity to get to know you, to learn how strong you really are, to depend on no one but you for your happiness . . . you will realize that a little loneliness goes a long way in creating a richer, deeper, more vibrant and colorful you."
— Mandy Hale, *The Single Woman: Life, Love, and a Dash of Sass.*

Why didn't the skeleton go to the dance?
It had no body to go with.

With vision, be on guard

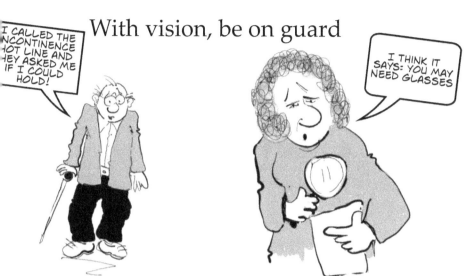

A woman walks into an optician to return a pair of spectacles that she purchased for her husband a week before. The assistant asks, "What seems to be the problem, Madam?"

The woman replies, "I'm returning these spectacles I bought for my husband. He's still not seeing things my way."

In the years after you turn 60, a number of eye diseases may develop that can change your vision permanently, according to the American Optometric Association. The earlier these problems are detected and treated, the more likely you can retain good vision.

The following are some vision disorders to be aware of:

Age-related macular degeneration (AMD) is an eye disease that affects the macula (the center of the light-sensitive retina at the back of the eye) and causes central vision loss. Although small, the macula is the part of the retina that allows us to see fine detail and colors. Activities like reading, driving, watching TV and recognizing faces all require good central vision provided by the macula. While macular degeneration decreases central vision, peripheral or side vision remains unaffected.

Cataracts are cloudy or opaque areas in the normally clear lens of the eye. Depending upon their size and location, they can interfere with normal vision. Usually cataracts develop in both eyes, but one may be worse than the other. Cataracts can cause blurry vision, decreased contrast sensitivity, dulling of colors and increased sensitivity to glare.

Diabetic retinopathy is a condition that occurs in people with diabetes. It is the result of progressive damage to the tiny blood vessels that nourish the retina. These damaged blood vessels leak blood and other fluids that cause retinal tissue to swell and cloud vision. The condition usually affects both eyes.

Dry eye is a condition in which a person produces too few or poor-quality tears. Tears maintain the health of the front surface of the eye and provide clear vision. Dry eye is a common and often chronic problem, particularly in older adults.

Glaucoma is a group of eye diseases characterized by damage to the optic nerve resulting in vision loss. People with a family history of glaucoma, African Americans and older adults have a higher risk of developing the disease. Glaucoma is often painless and can have no symptoms. Over time, it can take away peripheral vision.

Retinal detachment is a tearing or separation of the retina from the underlying tissue. Retinal detachment most often occurs spontaneously due to changes to the gel-like vitreous fluid that fills the back of the eye. Other causes include trauma to the eye or head, health problems like advanced diabetes, and inflammatory eye disorders. If not treated promptly, it can cause permanent vision loss.

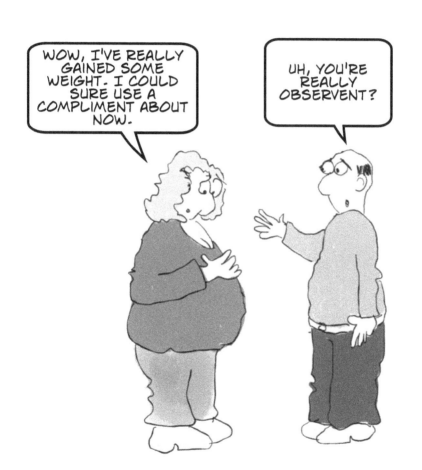

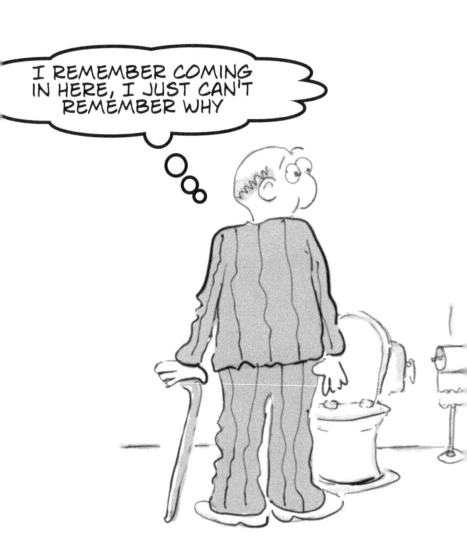

Kegeling for better control

Two ladies are chatting at the supermarket. One says, "I've given up the search for Mind Over Matter. Now I'm focusing on Mind Over Bladder."

Women over the age of fifty are apt to have urinary incontinence. Pelvic muscles weaken and become unable to control the bladder. Men with enlarged prostate glands also often have incontinence. People with the condition should check with their doctors about the many available treatments.

To help improve bladder control . . .

Avoid drinking excess amounts of diuretics.

Don't smoke. It irritates the bladder.

Wearing protective devices such as absorbent products, underwear, and adult diapers or using bed pads can also help manage the problem.

A magnesium supplement may prove helpful.

Kegel exercises strengthen the muscles that are squeezed when trying to stop urinating midstream. The exercises strengthen the pelvic floor muscle controlling urine flow and help hold pelvic organs in place. Here's how to develop the muscles:

For three seconds squeeze the muscles you use to stop urinating, then relax for three seconds. (Your stomach and thigh muscles should not tighten when you do this.) Add one second per week until you can squeeze for ten seconds each time.

Repeat this exercise ten to fifteen times per session. Try to do this at least three times a day. Don't do this exercise when urinating. If there's no change after three months, talk to your doctor.

Men may discover an exercise bonus of better orgasms and improved erections, and women often improve their posture.

An elderly couple visits their doctor for a checkup. The man goes in first.

"How're you doing?" asks the doctor.

"Pretty good," the old man says. "I'm eating well, and I'm still in control of my bowels and bladder. In fact, when I get up at night to pee, the good Lord turns the light on for me.'

The doctor ignores that last statement, and goes into the next room to check on the man's wife.

"How're you feeling?" he asks.

"I'm doing well," she says. "I have lots of energy and I'm not feeling any pain."

The doctor says, "That's nice. It sounds like you two are both doing well. One thing though—your husband said that when he gets up to pee at night, the Lord turns the light on for him. Do you have any idea what he means?"

"Oh, no," says the woman, "He's peeing in the refrigerator again."

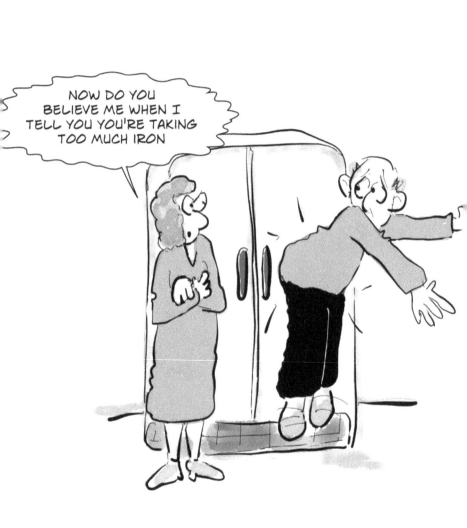

Medication upson downs

Tom Antion offers these drug-related observations:

I stopped taking tranquilizers. I was starting to be nice to people I didn't even want to talk to.

Mom takes so many iron tablets the only time she feels good is when she's facing magnetic north. My brothers are fighting over her mineral rights.

Hypochondriac: Someone who takes different pills than you do.

If laughter was the best medicine, doctors would find a way to charge for it.

Costrophobia: Fear of rising drug prices.

Diet tranquilizer: You don't lose weight, but you really don't care.

Prescription drug addiction is a disease most often caused by the misuse of drugs, according to Drugwatch, which offers the following information:
Some people become addicted to drugs even if taken as prescribed. Doctors prescribe them based on age, weight, family history, other medications being taken, and medical history. If doctors lack accurate or complete information, they may incorrectly prescribe the drug.
Biologically, addiction occurs because of the way drugs affect the brain. The brain receives information, processes it and then

communicates it to other parts of the body. It's made up of multiple parts that perform different functions. Drugs interfere with the way the brain works, and long-term use of certain drugs can cause permanent changes.

Different drugs affect the brain in different ways, but they all affect the way nerve cells in the brain communicate. Some drugs mimic chemicals in the brain, and others over-stimulate the "reward" part of the brain. For example, opioids imitate a neurotransmitter that affects the brain's nerve cells, causing them to send unusual communication to different parts of the body. Stimulants over-stimulate the "reward" part of the brain, causing a neurotransmitter called dopamine to be released. Dopamine produces happy feelings. When too much is released, it can cause a sense of euphoria or a "high."

It's these feelings that lead to addiction. The brain remembers things that make us happy and programs itself to want to do those things again. When people misuse prescription drugs, the brain programs itself to want to continue that behavior, but it releases less dopamine each time. Decreased dopamine production causes withdrawal and an increased tolerance to drugs.

Long-term misuse of drugs can lead to drastic changes in the way the brain works.

A woman went into the doctor's office and said, "I'd like to have some birth control pills."

Taken aback, the doctor thought for a minute then said, "Excuse me, Mrs. Jones, but you're 75 years old. What possible use could you have for birth control pills?"

The woman responded, "They help me sleep better."

The doctor thought some more and continued, "How in the world do birth control pills help you to sleep?"

The woman said, "I put them in my granddaughter's orange juice."

What's in a name?

Here are some team names for a senior walking race: Behind the Times; Keep on Truckin,' Too Old to Run, and Team Huff and Puff.

Judith Graham had called Ann Fishman, president of Generational Targeted Marketing, with a simple question. "What language should be used in talking about people age 65 and older? Seniors? The elderly? Older adults? Something else?"

Marketers, Fishman noted, make it point to address potential customers' "stage of life" and "lifestyle," but never talk about their age.

Graham decided to conduct a random, unscientific survey by calling a few mostly past-middle-age experts and asking what they thought. Here are their responses:

Harry Moody, 67, director of academic affairs for AARP, said, "What's going on is we have a problem with the subject itself. Everyone wants to live longer, but no one wants to be old. Personally, I tend to use the term 'older people' because it's the least problematic. Everyone is older than someone else."

Jane Glen Haas, 74, nationally syndicated newspaper columnist, said, "Don't call anyone 'elderly.' I associate that with people with physical disabilities who need constant care. 'Senior citizens' is a term coined in the late 1930s for people who needed a place to go, senior centers, to have a good lunch. To me, it implies somewhat impoverished older people, not the way people want to think of themselves. I guess 'older people' is best. I suppose if you had to call me something, I'd prefer that it be 'writer' or 'an older writer.''

Dr. John Rowe, 67, chairman of the MacArthur Foundation Research Network on an Aging Society and a professor of health policy at Columbia University, said, "People who study this talk about the 'young-old,' roughly age 65 to 75, and the 'old-old,' a group that tends to have more physical needs. The problem with terms like 'the elderly' or 'seniors' is that they lump these two groups together, and none of the young-old want to be identified with the old-old. When I'm talking about individuals, then I say 'older person.' Personally, I prefer the term 'senior,' but the fact is no one calls me that because no one thinks I'm that old."

"In general," said Judith Graham, "I'd prefer to refer to people as they'd like to be called, but I don't know what that is."

Ina Jaffe, an award-winning NPR correspondent, quoted Ann Fishman during a radio segment on what to call old people. "Since the early 20th century, we've added at least 30 years to the average life expectancy, and the language just hasn't caught up with that," Jaffe said.

But maybe this will stick: "There's a term I found—wouldn't you know—on Twitter," Jaffe said. "Recently, someone I follow tweeted that she was buying tickets to a show in London, and instead of senior discount, they used the term 'super adult.'"

Some popular bumper stickers:

Fishmore Doolittle
Some of the sweetest music is played on the oldest fiddle
Retirement Planning Consultant
I'm not old. I'm extra crispy.
Enjoy life. It has an expiration date.

Steps to cope with stress

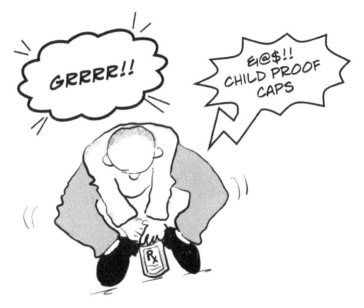

Stress is when you wake up screaming and you realize you haven't fallen asleep yet.

The American Heart Association suggests these ways to manage stress:

Positive self-talk. We all talk to ourselves; sometimes we talk out loud but usually we keep self-talk in our heads. It can be positive ("I can do this" or "Things will work out"). The thing to remember is forgo negative self-talk. To help you feel better, practice positive self-talk every day—in the car, at your desk, before you go to bed, or whenever you notice negative thoughts.

Try emergency stress stoppers when you're in a bind because of poor communication, too much work, and everyday hassles like standing in line. Emergency stress stoppers help you deal with stress on the spot. Try these:

> Count to 10 before you speak.
> Take three to five deep breaths.
> Walk away from the stressful situation, and say you'll handle it later.
> Go for a walk.
> Say "I'm sorry" if you make a mistake.
> Set your watch five minutes ahead to avoid the stress of being late.

When stress makes you feel bad, do something that makes you feel good. Doing things you enjoy is a natural way to fight back. Go for a drive, chat with a friend, or read a good book.

Try to do at least one thing every day that you enjoy, even if you only do it for 15 minutes. Start an art project. Take up a hobby, new or old. Read a favorite book, short story, magazine, or newspaper. Have coffee or a meal with friends. Play tennis, sew, or knit. Listen to music during or after you practice relaxation.

Relaxation can calm the tension in your mind and body. Some good forms are yoga, tai chi, and meditation. Deep breathing also is a form of relaxation you can learn and practice at home. Try to devote five to 10 minutes every day for deep breathing or another form of relaxation.

Q. What's the difference between "anxiety" and "panic"?

A. "Anxiety" is when, for the first time, you can't do it the second time. "Panic" is when, for the second time, you can't do it the first time.

Problems on a weighty matter

A woman at the doctor's office said to the doctor, "Doctor, I beg of you, please prescribe me something immediately to reduce my weight. My husband has given me a wonderful birthday present, and I can't get into it."

Doctor: "Just visit here tomorrow, and I'll give you a prescription. Then you will soon be able to wear your wonderful new dress."

Lady: "Who said anything about a dress? I am talking of a car."

During the past 30 years, the proportion of older adults who are obese has doubled, according to one study. In spite of the increase, the majority of older adults are not obese and continue to lead active and healthy lives.

Currently, however, the number of people over 65 years of age in the U.S. is projected to rise from 12 percent (35 million) to 20 percent (71 million) by 2030. These substantial increases among older adults suggest that obesity among older Americans is likely to become a greater problem in the future. By 2000, the prevalence of obesity in people 50 to 69 years of age was 22.9 percent, and, for those above 70, about 15 percent.

As the aging population increases, so too will the number of obesity-related chronic conditions, such as arthritis, diabetes, hypertension, and heart disease. Healthy eating habits and physical activity are key aspects of achieving a healthy weight, experts say. The loss of weight and lack of nutrition associated with a chronic illness is referred to as cachexia. Unexplained, unintentional weight loss is often a result of illness and should be evaluated by a health-care professional.

Alfred was so fat when he stepped on the scale it said, "To be continued."

"I'm not overweight, I'm just nine inches too short."
—Shelley Winters

Many are getting in deeper

If you think no one cares about you, try missing a debt payment.

More seniors are carrying debt into retirement than ever before, according to the National Council on Aging. It reported that Survey of Consumer Finances, found that senior households with any debt increased from nearly 50 percent in 1989 to just over 61 percent in 2013.

Median total debt for older adult households with debt was $40,900 in 2013—more than double the 2001 amount.

Increasingly, medical debt poses the most significant barrier to economic well-being, the survey found. More than 84 percent of people aged 65+ are coping with at least one chronic condition, and often more as they age.

A study in the Journal of General Internal Medicine revealed that out-of-pocket medical expenditures in the five years prior to an individual's death totaled more than $38,000, leaving one in four seniors approaching bankruptcy.

Another common source of debt among senior households is credit cards. In 2001, approximately 27 percent of senior households held credit card balances; by 2013, more than 32 percent did.

Living on Earth is expensive, but it does include a free trip around the sun every year.   —Unknown

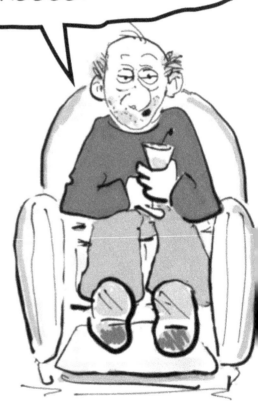

Dealing with painful moments

A man sits down on a bus seat by a priest. The man's tie is askew, his face red with lipstick, and a bottle of booze protrudes from his pocket. He glances at his newspaper, then turns to the priest and says, "Father, can you tell me what causes arthritis?"

"Oftentimes it's a result of loose living, cheap women and too much alcohol."

"Well, imagine that," the man says. He begins reading again.

The priest ponders a moment, nudges the man and says, "Forgive me. I shouldn't have been so candid. Have you had arthritis very long?"

"Nope, Father. I don't have it. I just noticed in the paper that the Pope does."

The Mayo Clinic staff says you can find out what will work best for you about easing the pain of arthritis and other conditions with exercise, medication and stress reduction. Here are some of the clinic's do's and don'ts to help you figure it out:

Talk to your doctor about your symptoms, arthritis related or not. Provide information about your medical conditions and medications, including over-the-counter items and supplements. Ask your doctor for a clear definition of the type of arthritis you have. Determine if any of your joints are already damaged.

Do some gentle exercise in the evening; you'll feel less stiff in the morning. When you're watching TV, reading or working at your desk, adjust your position frequently. Periodically tilt your neck from side to side, change the position of your hands, and bend and stretch your legs. Pace yourself. Take breaks so that you don't overuse a single joint and cause more pain. Stand and walk around every half-hour or so.

Lifestyle changes are important for easing pain. Being over-weight can increase complications of arthritis and contribute to its pain. Gradual weight loss is often the most effective method of weight management. Quit smoking.

When you have arthritis, movement can decrease your pain, improve your range of motion, strengthen your muscles and in-crease your endurance. Choose the right kinds of activities— those that build the muscles around your joints but don't dam-age the joints themselves. A physical or occupational therapist can help. Focus on stretching, range-of-motion exercises and gradual progressive strength training. Include walking, cycling or water exercises, to improve your mood and help control your weight. Avoid running, jumping, tennis, high-impact aerobics, and repeating the same movement, such as a tennis serve, again and again.

Many types of medications are available for arthritis. Most are relatively safe, but no medication is completely free of side effects. Talk with your doctor to formulate a medication plan.

Over-the-counter pain medications, such as acetaminophen (Tylenol, others) or ibuprofen (Advil, Motrin IB, others), can help relieve occasional pain triggered by activity your muscles and joints aren't used to - such as gardening after a winter indoors. Topical analgesics. Cream containing capsaicin may be applied to skin over a painful joint to relieve pain. Use alone or with oral medication.

How to get the sleep you need

Laugh and the world laughs with you; snore, and you sleep alone.   —Anthony Burgess

People who say they sleep like a baby usually don't have one.
  —Leo J. Burke

People who snore always fall asleep first.
  —Unknown Author

A day without a nap is like a cupcake without frosting.
  —Terri Guillemets

"Often, the first thing students tell me when they start a daily yoga practice is that they sleep better," says Susi Amendola in the *Ornish Living* newsletter. "They report falling asleep easier and sleeping more deeply because yoga has tools to combat insomnia and sleep issues."

Here are some of her favorite tips on sleep:

• Walk slowly without the "push" of exercise. This calms the nervous system and allows the energy of the mind to gently inhabit the spaces of the body.

• Rest with your legs up the wall. This brings fresh blood back to the heart so the heart doesn't have to pump so hard. In turn, it lowers blood pressure and heart rate.

• Deep relaxation during the day allows physical and mental tensions to gently unwind and dissipate.

• Do alternate nostril breathing 10 minutes before bedtime. This calms the nervous system and quiets the mind. It's also used to prepare the mind for meditation.

• Try turning off all technology at least one hour prior to sleeping. Keeping the room dark in general can promote good sleep.

• Avoid caffeine after noon. If you are sensitive to caffeine, you may not be able to drink any without it interfering with sleep patterns. Even dark chocolate and green tea can be too stimulating.

• Going to bed and getting up at the same time each day helps the body find a healthy rhythm. This can be an important key to good sleep and good health.

• Reading something uplifting right before sleep can be just the right way to set the mind at ease and support a sense of security and peace so the mind can gently drift off.

• Treat yourself to a warm bedtime drink.

• Reduce added stimulation such as heated conversations, spicy foods, heavy exercise, cleaning, excessive work, and that late-night movie murder mystery.

I'm so good at sleeping I can do it with my eyes closed.

Looking for new rules?

From *The New Official Rules*, a book of new rules, laws, and maxims assembled by Paul Dickson:

The older I get, the better I used to be.　　—Quote in Bob Levey's *Washington Post* column.

I'd rather have a free bottle in front of me than a prefrontal lobotomy.　　—Fred Allen

Only Robinson Crusoe had everything done by Friday.
　　—C.A. Munro

You're either too young or old enough to know better, but you're never the right age.　　—Peggy McCormick

The older you get, the easier it is to resist temptation, but the harder it is to find.　　—Joseph H. Humpert, MD.

It matters not so much whether you do something well or badly, but how you get out of doing it honestly.
　　—Kurt Anderson

A writer for *Upgrade Reality* offers these rules to live by:

Do unto others as you want others to do to you.

Treasure your body for it is the vessel that guides you through your life. Make it a habit to eat a healthy and natural diet, exercise, and get plenty of sleep. Also, avoid stress.

Be honest and always tell the truth. However, there will be times when a white lie is necessary to prevent hurting people's feelings.

Success requires hard work, persistence and a little creativity. Don't hope for a quick fix, but be prepared for the long haul. Keep learning and never give up.

Make a difference to at least one other person's life.

Admit when you're wrong and apologize.

You can learn something from everyone.

Don't be scared; go through life as fearlessly as possible. Ask yourself, "Would you rather play it safe to not risk failure or would you rather risk failure to really live and do what your heart tells you should do?"

Smile and laugh every single day.

Count your blessings and be thankful for all the good things in your life. As the saying goes: The past is history, the future is a mystery, and right now is a gift; that's why they call it the "present."

It should come as no surprise that agencies that deal with older adults have developed a few maxims from assisting seniors over the years. For example:

Some relatives, friends or even caretakers who volunteer to handle bill-paying for an older person will generously pay themselves.

The investment of time and effort in enabling seniors to remain living independently pays healthy dividends.

To foil that rascal Al Z. Heimer, try new things, socialize and exercise.

If you like to shop, dispose of two things for every one you buy.

When you falter or stall, give your Area Agency on Aging a call.

What you need for healthiness

Some cause happiness wherever they go; others whenever they go.   —Oscar Wilde

Health is the greatest of all possessions; a pale cobbler is better than a sick king.
    —Bickerstaff

What is the key to happiness? Some believe it's being rich, others think its stardom. In a study by the Harvard Study of Adult Development, one other factor dominates. Robert J. Waldinger, a Harvard Medical School professor, says that the study, which began 75 years ago, found that positive relationships count the most. "Good relationships keep us happier and healthier. Period," Waldinger says. "It turns out that people who are more socially connected to family, to friends, to community, are happier. They're physically healthier and they live longer than people who are less well connected. And the experience of loneliness turns out to be toxic."

It isn't necessarily that people needed to be in a committed relationship. "It's the quality of your close relationships that matters," he said. "It turns out that living in the midst of conflict is really bad for our health."

The study enlisted 724 men from the Boston area—268 sophomores from Harvard College and 456 inner-city teenagers—and followed them as they aged. Nearly 60 of them are still alive and participating in the study. Waldinger says the researchers are even starting to study the 2,000 children of these men.

A relationship is like a house. When a light bulb burns out you do not go out and buy a new house, you fix the bulb.

Steering clear of abuse

Hospital regulations require a wheelchair for patients being discharged. However, while working as a student nurse, I found one elderly gentleman already dressed and sitting on the bed with a suitcase at his feet, who insisted he didn't need my help to leave the hospital. After a chat about rules being rules, he reluctantly let me wheel him to the elevator. On the way down I asked him if his wife was meeting him. "I don't know," he said "She's still upstairs in the bathroom changing out of her hospital gown."   —Anonymous

About five million elders are abused each year, according to research by the National Council on Aging. It cites one study estimating that only one in 14 cases of abuse are reported to authorities.

In almost 90 percent of elder abuse and neglect incidents, the perpetrator is a family member, the NCOA found. Two thirds of perpetrators are adult children or spouses.

Social isolation and mental impairment (such as dementia or Alzheimer's disease) are two abuse factors. Nearly half of those with dementia experienced abuse or neglect. Interpersonal violence also occurs at disproportionately higher rates among adults with disabilities.

The warning signs of elder abuse include physical abuse, neglect, or mistreatment: bruises, pressure marks, broken bones, abrasions, and burns, the NCOA reported. It also found that emotional abuse is characterized by unexplained withdrawal from normal activities, a sudden change in alertness, or unusual depression; strained or tense relationships; frequent arguments between the caregiver and older adult.

Sudden changes in financial situations suggest a problem.

While likely underreported, financial abuse costs older Americans $2.9 billion per year. Yet, financial exploitation is self-reported at rates higher than emotional, physical, and sexual abuse or neglect. Elders who have been abused have a 300 percent higher risk of death when compared to those who have not been mistreated, said NCOA.

Older adults can stay safe by seeking professional help for drug, alcohol, and depression concerns. With a power of attorney or a living will, they can address health care decisions now to avoid confusion and family problems later. Staying active in the community and connected with friends and family will decrease social isolation, which has been connected to elder abuse.

Other NCOA tips include:

Posting and opening your own mail.
Not giving personal information over the phone.
Using direct deposit for all checks.
Having your own phone.
Reviewing your will periodically.
Knowing your rights.

If you engage the services of a paid or family caregiver, you have the right to voice your preferences and concerns. If you live in a nursing home, call your Long Term Care Ombudsman. The ombudsman is your advocate and has the power to intervene.

"Poor old fool," thought the well-dressed gentleman as he watched an old man fish in a puddle outside a pub. So he invited the old man inside for a drink. As they sipped their whiskeys, the gentleman thought he'd humor the old man and asked, "So how many have you caught today?"

The old man replied, "You're the eighth."

Where to find the answers

A wise man once said, "I look to the future because that's where I'm going to spend the rest of my life."

George Burns used this line during shows when he was in his nineties. In his book, *Wisdom of the Nineties,* he said, "Being old isn't such a handicap. In some ways it's a help. You can't do as much and there may be things you can't do as well, but nobody expects you to. Old-timers don't have to come in first. They get credit for just showing up. And if they're out there making a real effort, they've got everyone pulling for them."

Many older adults can feel fortunate because they have folks pulling for them. In the U.S. there are 629 Area Agencies on Aging, for example. Contact your local agency for expert advice on your problem, and obtain contact information about firms and agencies that meet your needs. Your senior center and associations dealing with challenges such as Alzheimer's also are sources of helpful information.

George Burns often offered helpful information, such as, "Happiness is having a large, loving, caring, close-knit family in another city." He could wax poetic. "How beautifully leaves grow old. How full of light and color are their last days." In celebration of Burns' 99th birthday in 1995, Los Angeles renamed a street "Gracie Allen Drive." It connects with a short street that is named for him. Burns was present at the unveiling ceremony where he quipped, "It's good to be here at the corner of Burns and Allen. At my age, it's good to be anywhere!"

Sayings that can help:

The only way to have a friend is to be one.
— Ralph Waldo Emerson

You cannot shake hands with a clenched fist.
— Indira Gandhi

You must be the change you wish to see in the world.
— Mahatma Gandhi

A bowl belongs to whoever needs it.
— A Native American saying

Without memory, there is no healing; without forgiveness, there is no future.   — Desmond Tutu

Wise men talk because they have something to say. Fools talk because they have to say something.   — Plato

Beauty is in the eye of the beer holder.   —Anon

Put yourself on autopilot

There's an old story that illustrates intuitive talent:

One day, three men were walking through a jungle when they came across a rapidly raging river. They had no idea how to cross. The first man decided to pray: "Please, God, give me the strength to cross this river." Quickly he grew great muscles in his arms and legs, and he swam across the river in a few hours, nearly drowning twice.

The second man saw this and he prayed, "Please, God, give me the strength and the tools to cross this river." A boat appeared, and he guided it across the river in an hour, nearly capsizing twice.

The third man saw this and prayed, "Please, God, give me the strength, the tools and the intelligence to cross this river." Immediately he turned into a woman. She looked at the map, walked upstream a hundred yards, and crossed over the bridge to the other side.

"Intuition is a natural mental ability, strongly associated with experience," says Roy Rowan, author of *The Intuitive Manager*. It heightens as we grow older, he believes.

As the years go by "we've accumulated life experience, a knowledge of other people, a sense of ourselves," he says. "Most important, we have the wisdom and courage to act on our instincts."

In Lauraine Snelling's book, *100 Good Things that Happen as You Grow Older*, she quotes therapist Gail Grundon: "I find and use my intuition in relationships with some of my friends and my daughter. I always knew when she was in trouble and have learned to call a friend when her name comes to mind insistently. I'm always glad when I listen to these promptings, and I've been sorry when I didn't."

Just what is intuition? It's when your brain goes on autopilot, says Hara Morano in *Psychology Today*. The brain is performing its actions of processing information outside of your awareness that it's operating. For example:

You walk down a street, get lost in thought, and find yourself at your destination without awareness of the processes that got you there.

"There is no substitute for gathering information about any task or situation before us," she writes. "But neither should we be afraid of not knowing every reason why we feel the way we do in every situation."

Mark Twain wasn't in doubt during his discussion about polygamy with a Mormon acquaintance. Frustrated, the Mormon said, "Can you tell me of a single passage of Scripture wherein polygamy is forbidden?"

"Certainly," Twain replied. "No man can serve two masters."

The value of choices

Ed Fisher and Jane Thomas Noland chose *What's Funny About Growing Old?* as the title of their book. It's a blend of his cartoons and her observations, such as, "Alice is determined to stay young at all costs. She buys only foods with preservatives." Under the title "Rose-colored bifocals" is this bit of wisdom: "The older you are, the smarter you were as a kid."

The cover's cartoon shows an elderly man who asks his wife, "What are you wearing-Chanel No. 5? Moonlight Musk? Love Mist?" She replies, "Vicks."

In the preface, Noland states, "Two things are absolutely essential in order to face the adventure of growing older: a healthy spirituality and a quick, robust sense of humor."

We can benefit by choosing to laugh at many of our situations and surroundings, she adds.

A Hopi Indian poem influenced both Lorrie and Chesley "Sully" Sullenberger. It goes like this:

There is a river flowing now very fast,
It is so great and swift that there are those who will be afraid,
They will try to hold onto the shore.
They will feel they are torn apart and will suffer greatly.
Know the river has its destination.
The elders say we must let go of the shore,
push off into the middle of the river.
Keep our eyes open, and our heads above water.

The poem helps the Sulllenbergers recognize that everyone must find the courage to leave the shore."That means leaving the crutch of our lifelong complaints and resentments, or our unhappiness over our upbringing or our bodies or whatever," says Captain Sullenberger in his book, *Highest Duty*. "It means no longer focusing negative energy on things beyond our control. It means looking beyond the safety of the familiar."

The concept is a reminder, he says, that "Our lives are a combination of what we can control, what we can't, and the results of choices we make."

As we grow older there may come the time when the challenges of daily living can benefit from a care manager's assessment that enables a senior to continue living independently. Perhaps the task of bill paying requires help that a fiduciary or money manager also can provide. Other choices that seniors make, with guidance from professionals like these, include financial decisions that protect their assets when impatient offspring believe they're entitled to them now.

By choosing the middle of the river, seniors continue their social ties, take part in local or senior center's activities, and lend a hand to those in need. They do, indeed, keep their eyes open and their heads above water.

Jane Thomas Noland puts it this way:

As you stand by the fridge's open door,
Letting all its cold pour out, you
Wonder—did you already eat your lunch?
Or are you just about to?

Targeting one, zero, zero

Despite our love of candy and fast food, the number of Americans who will live to be 100 years or older will increase dramatically. In 2010 there were 53,000 centenarians in the United States, and I have driven behind every single one.
—Jimmy Kimmel

One of the growing segments of the U.S. population is the group whose members top 100 years old. The U.S. Census Bureau predicts one million Americans will be 100 years old or older by 2040. Do you have a chance of reaching or passing that age? It may take some lifestyle changes, plus tips from researchers who have been studying the centenarians.

"Older doesn't mean sicker," says Thomas Perls, MD, founder and director of the New England Centenarian Study, which was created in 1994 with Boston University help. "The vast majority of individuals we study live independently for most of their lives, and we have found that the older you live usually means the healthier you've lived."

The work of Dr. Perls and studies on varied activities may lead to improved life spans. "We have a great deal of power over our longevity, and the decisions we make every day contribute to our life expectancy," he says. "I know that after working with centenarians, I have changed my habits. I lost thirty pounds and think twice before grabbing a high-fat snack at the checkout counter."

Posit Science, a provider of brain-training software, offers this rather unusual tip:

Exercise your peripheral vision. Sit in a place outside your house, such as on a park bench or in a café. Stare straight ahead and don't move your eyes. Concentrate on everything you can see without moving your eyes, including items in your peripheral vision. When you have finished, write a list of everything you saw. Then try again and see if you can add to your list. The reason: scientists have shown that the neurotransmitter acetylcholine, which is crucial to focus and memory, falls off with memory loss and is almost absent in Alzheimer's patients. This activity should help you reinvigorate the controlled release of acetylcholine in your brain through a useful visual memory task.

A 105-year-old in the New England Centenarian study quipped to researchers. "You know the best thing about being over 100 is you no longer have to worry about peer pressure — you no longer have any peers left."

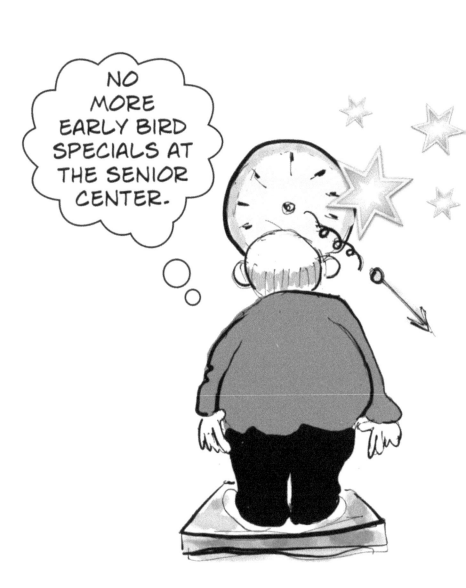

Remodeling your brain

The way I see it . . . If you need both of your hands for whatever it is you're doing, then your brain should probably be in on it too.   —Ellen DeGeneres

The steps of improving the brain at first appear easy. If you watch your diet, exercise, socialize, and manage stress, you can extend the telomeres, those small yet vital tips on your chromosomes. People with improved telomeres not only enhance their memory and cognition, they live five years longer than those with shortened chromosomes, based on recent research.

Linda Fodrini-Johnson, founder of Eldercare Services, outlined the steps and research results during a workshop in Walnut Creek, California. Her tips for a healthier diet include whole foods, plant-based protein, fruits, vegetables, and refined carbohydrates. Basic aerobic exercise, such as a thirty-minute walk six days a week, keep you fit while boosting telomeres.

As a sidelight on the need for social activity, she said that two million Americans over the age of sixty-five live in isolation. Weekly support group sessions prove helpful to many who lack interaction, she added.

Meditation helps many people cope with stress. Some advisors recommend one hour a day, but she finds half that amount suffices. Yoga, mindfulness, brief pauses, and breathing breaks help maintain one's calmness. She cited key factors that inhibit the brain, including inflammation, illnesses such as arthritis, anxiety, unhealthy foods, infections, too much alcohol, and smoking.

One key culprit, Fodrini-Johnson said, is a low vitamin D level. "Call your doctor and have it checked during your next lab visit," she suggested. People with low levels may experience problems with their hearts, joints, and cognition. A recommended level is at least 1,000 units per day.

She led those in attendance in a "4-7-8" breathing exercise that serves as a tranquilizer for the nervous system. The first step is exhaling with a "whoosh" sound. Close your mouth and inhale through the nose to a count of four. Hold your breath for a count of seven. Exhale through the mouth with another "whoosh" for a count of eight. Do this twice a day.

Her brain remodeling tips included brain exercises, video games such as Lumosity, crossword puzzles, Sudoku, and engaging in varied activities. People benefit when, at the end of the day, they recall three things they're grateful for, she added.

It's not that I'm so smart, it's just that I stay with problems longer.   —Alfred Einstein

Keeping perspective

Setting goals is the first step in turning the invisible into the visible.   —Tony Robbins

In his book, *Rules for Aging*, Roger Rosenblatt tells about the man who ordered a freezer from the appliance store. The sales rep promised delivery between 1 and 4 p.m., but it didn't arrive. The home owner phoned and angrily demanded to know where the freezer was. Told that it definitely would be delivered the following day between 8 and 11 a.m., he remarked to his wife, "They had better do it this time or else."

The store failed to deliver the freezer again, and the man was livid. He called the store manager and yelled into the phone. He called his lawyer. "You're making too much of this," his wife said. "The freezer will get here eventually. You are really starting to annoy me."

He told her to shut up, and asked whose side was she on, anyway. Then he called the store again. This time he threatened to kill the store manager. The manager called his lawyer.

The wife, realizing she had married a maniac, called her lawyer.

In the end, the transaction cost the man his wife, $250,000 in damages, and the house in which he had planned to install the freezer. The moral, says Rosenblatt, winner of two George Polk Awards, a Peabody, and an Emmy, is: remember the freezer.

"Every one of life's little mishaps can be kept in perspective if one focuses on one's original goal—in this case to acquire a freezer."

With ordinary talent and extraordinary perseverance, all things are attainable.   —Thomas Buxton

Benefits of a perfect blendship

Betty White's book, *If You Ask Me, and Of Course You Won't*, includes some interesting observations, such as:

"As the years add up, I am so grateful for the good health I have been blessed with, and I don't ever take it for granted for a second.

"I make it a point to never let my weight vary more than five pounds in either direction. I wear glasses to read or to drive.

"I have a two-level house and a bad memory, so all those trips up and downstairs take care of my exercise . . . As to my hair, I have no idea what color it really is, and I never intend to find out."

The TV star, who turned 93 in 2015, also said, "Friendship takes time and energy if it's going to work. You can luck into something great, but it doesn't last if you don't give it proper appreciation. Friendship can be so comfortable, but nurture it—don't take it for granted."

Studies have shown that friendships reduce stress. This can lower the risk of a terminal illness. Good friends also boost one's happiness level, and that has health benefits. To establish a friendship, strike up a conversation with someone at a play, the senior center, church, or other gathering. Arrange a get-together at lunch or a mutually enjoyable event and pursue your interests.

Winnie the Pooh remarked, "You can't stay in your corner of the forest waiting for others to come to you. You have to go to them sometimes."

It's a good idea, too, to remember what John Leonard said: "It takes a long time to grow an old friend."

Here are some more of Betty White's quotes on the topic:

Keep the other person's well being in mind when you feel an attack of soul-purging truth coming on.

All creatures must learn to coexist. That's why the brown bear and the field mouse can share their lives in harmony. Or course, they can't mate or the mice would explode.

I just make it my business to get along with people so I can have fun. It's that simple.

White also recalls, "My mother always used to say, 'The older you get, the better you get. Unless you're a banana.'"

Weight loss ideas

Bathroom scale tips:

1. Weigh yourself fully clothed after dinner and again the next morning without clothes and before breakfast, because it's nice to see how much weight you've lost overnight.

2. Never weigh yourself with wet hair.

3. When weighing, remove everything, including eyeglasses. In this case, blurred vision is an asset. Don't forget to remove jewelry as it could weigh as much as a pound!

4. Buy only cheap scales, never the medical kind. Accuracy is the enemy and high quality scales are very accurate.

5. Always go to the bathroom first.

6. Weigh yourself after a haircut, this is good for up to half a pound of hair (hopefully).

7. Exhale with all your might BEFORE stepping onto the scale. (Air has weight, right?)

"The biggest mistake people over 50 make is believing it's inevitable to gain weight as we age," says Deborah Orlick Levy, a registered dietician and health and nutrition consultant for Carrington Farms. "Implementing healthful strategies can result in better overall health and weight control." Various gimmicks and dubious rapid weight loss methods may provide weight loss, but only temporarily. "For both sexes, you are going to have to fight harder to lose those extra pounds," says Dr. Brian Quebbemann, a bariatric surgeon and founder of the N.E.W. Program in Newport Beach, California.

Here's how:

"You'll need to up your exercise routine or start one if you're not currently working out," says Dr. Levy. "Not only for overall health, but to shed those excess pounds by increasing metabolism and muscle mass." Eat less, says Dr. Quebbemann. Some people experience reduced appetite as they age, but not always. "For those people who do not experience a decrease in appetite, it is even more important to maintain your activity level." It also helps to eat fewer calories by filling up on lean protein, whole grains, fruits and vegetables, and avoid foods lacking in nutrients, says Dr. Levy. Dr. Quebbemann advises men to get annual check-ups to ensure their testosterone levels are not abnormally decreased.

Men and women should also get tested for insulin resistance. It may result in elevated blood sugar (often called pre-diabetes) and more rapid accumulation of abdominal fat. Medications to balance blood sugar can result in sustained weight loss. It's total calories that count; the timing of when you eat is less important. "The best solution, of course, is to simply pay more attention to your diet, and be more responsible in avoiding those extra calories throughout the day," says Dr. Quebbemann.

No diet will remove all the fat from your body because the brain is entirely fat. Without a brain, you might look good, but all you could do is run for public office. —George Bernard Shaw

Dealing with irritation

Your voice is like brain sandpaper.   —Eileen Miller

George Burns wrote a chapter about irritation and aggravation in his book, *Dr. Burns' Prescription for Happiness* published in 1984. "To me, irritation is something that makes your skin red," he stated. "Aggravation is paying the pharmacy $12.50 for something to cure the irritation, and when you get the bottle home you can't open it. Right there we have one of the major aggravations of 20th Century America. Nothing opens. Jars are impossible. Peanut butter, jam, pickles, those lids are on to stay."

He tried the technique of dousing the lid of a mayonnaise jar with warm water, then pounding it. "I pounded the lid on the kitchen sink, broke the jar, had mayonnaise all over the sink, but the lid stayed on." The worst of all, he said, are prescription bottles. "When they started making them child-proof, did it ever occur to them they were also making them senior-citizen-proof?" he asked.

"Dr." Burns acknowledged that exercise, meditation, and spas provide stress and tension relief for many, then added that these can also reduce the money in their wallets. As for his happiness prescription, he said, ". . .without fear of contradiction it's enjoying your work," while admitting those who are retired or rich may still be happy. "I don't understand them, but I know they're out there."

Most people do not listen with the intent to understand; they listen with the intent to reply.   —Stephen R. Covey

A̶BOOKS

ALIVE Book Publishing and ALIVE Publishing Group
are imprints of Advanced Publishing LLC,
3200 A Danville Blvd., Suite 204, Alamo, California 94507

Telephone: 925.837.7303 Fax: 925.837.6951
www.alivebookpublishing.com

CPSIA information can be obtained
at www.ICGtesting.com
Printed in the USA
FSHW010019110219
55529FS